Medical Marijuana

The Basic Principles For Cannabis Medicine

By Aaron Hammond

Version 2.2

Published by HMPL Publishing at KDP

Get to know your publisher and his work at:

http://happyhealthygreen.life

A personal note from the author

Ihave always been interested in cannabis and the medical benefits of marijuana. Writing this book and sharing information and insights about the, still controversial, substance known as 'cannabis' has been a pleasure.

The science is out there and clinical research does not lie. I am as much grateful as I am happy that you are reading these words. HMPL Publishing and I are dedicated to providing you with recent, accurate and justifiable facts that are backed up by more than mere words.

Let's make a change together and open up our eyes to the power of nature. I've released books about CBD, Hemp-oil, and cannabis extracts. I will continue to provide you with the best information and make it easy to understand.

In this book, I'd like to share information about cannabis and teach you the mechanics of cannabinoids; how these little compounds can have such a tremendous impact on our body and provide their many medicinal benefits.

Shortly, I will go over various important topics within the world of medical marijuana to inform you what is possible and get you up to date with everything related to the history of marijuana legalization.

In the future, we will shift focus to in-depth information, providing you with everything you need to know on cannabis, so make sure you get on par with the subject through our books!

With kind regards,
Aaron Hammond

solitary and utter responsibility of the recipient reader. Under no circumstances will any legal responsibility or blame be held against the publisher for any reparation, damage, or monetary loss due to the information herein, either directly or indirectly.

Respective authors own all copyrights not held by the publisher. The information herein is offered for informational purposes solely, and is universal as so. The presentation of the information is without contract or any type of guarantee assurance. The trademarks that are used are without any consent, and the publication of the trademark is without permission or backing by the trademark owner. All trademarks and brands within this book are for clarifying purposes only and are owned by the owners themselves, not affiliated with this document. We don't encourage any substance abuse and we cannot be held responsible for any partaking in illegal activities.

Aaron Hammond

Table of Contents

Cannabis: The Ins and Outs

C annabis is the generally accepted name for the plant *Cannabis sativa* L. This species is also referred to as marijuana and is a member of the hemp family. Even though "cannabis" and "hemp" are often used interchangeably, they are not exactly the same thing. "Hemp" refers to the varieties of *Cannabis sativa* L. that don't have psychoactive effects. In other words, all kinds of the cannabis plant that contain less than 1% THC content are technically "hemp."

When it comes to differentiating between hemp and marijuana, think of what purpose the plant was bred for. When cannabis is bred for fiber, industrial purposes, oils, ointments, or for any other use that is not intoxication, it is "hemp." "Marijuana" originated as a slang term for cannabis strains bred to be used for intoxication. These strains have tiny, potent "hairs" (trichomes) on the flowers and leaves that contain active compounds which produce various effects within the body. Keeping these differences straight can be confusing, so just remember that in their simplest terms marijuana causes a high and hemp does not. Both can be classified as cannabis.

Marijuana Stigma

The public certainly has mixed opinions about cannabis, especially the recreational variety. While a large part of the population seems to be pro-marijuana, there is major defense against it. In the United States as of 2017, only 8 states have legalized marijuana use - consuming, cultivating, or growing - for people 21 years and older. In addition to this kind of legalization in 8 states, there are 18 states that have decriminalized marijuana and 29 states that permit medical use.

However, there is still quite a bit of controversy over the cannabis plant in the US, especially among the older generation. This may be in part due to the timeline of marijuana. When the War on Drugs kicked off several decades ago, it stirred up a lot of intense feelings and political stances, which the older generation of today may not have let go. In 1986, President Reagan signed the Anti-Drug Abuse Act, which meant that drug-related crimes would now require mandatory sentences. The possession and selling of marijuana soon fell under federal penalty. Then in 1989, President Bush reignited the country's passion against drugs with a new "War on Drugs." His speech was aired on televisions nationwide. Millennials, on the other hand, have grown up in a society that holds less conservative opinions of marijuana overall, creating a massive divide between young and old adults. To this day, many conservatives still speak out against marijuana use. Those against it do everything in their power to create legislation that not only criminalizes recreational cannabis but places a stigma on medical marijuana as well.

Since 1970, cannabis has been listed as a Schedule 1 drug in the US. Schedule 1 drugs - which include heroin, LSD, ecstasy, and peyote - are defined as drugs "with no currently accepted medical use and a high potential for abuse." Many people have a problem with this, considering the positive attention marijuana has gotten in the medical field all over the world in recent research. In early 2017, a report published by the National Academies of Sciences, Engineering, and Medicine (NASEM) showed evidence that cannabis provides potent health benefits, including reducing chronic pain. As of today, this is the most popular reason that medical marijuana is requested by patients.

Why it is still classified as a Schedule 1 drug is hard to understand based on the wealth of research on its medical benefits, not to mention the lack of proof of marijuana toxicity or any potential risk of death (which other Schedule 1 drugs and even alcohol have all shown). It also does not possess symptoms of other "hard drugs" that are in the Schedule 1 category. Typical symptoms of smoking or ingesting marijuana include relaxation and sleepiness along with a "high" or mild euphoria. With higher amounts these symptoms expand to include dry mouth, redness of the eyes, reduced motor skills, and impaired short term memory. However, none of these effects are permanent. Only when laced or mixed with more dangerous drugs does marijuana cause more intense symptoms. It is even less harmful than alcohol, a substance that doesn't appear in the drug schedules at all. In a study that compared marijuana and 10 other drugs for its "potential of death" when being used in typical recreational fashion, marijuana was the least dangerous. Despite these findings, and the fact that most Americans do favor marijuana, there has been little headway made in government to reduce the restrictions. This is only intensifying the split in opinions because Schedule 1 drugs face more obstacles for being researched. Without the necessary research to provide more evidence that it provides medical benefits, convincing the rest of the American public of marijuana's innocence will prove very difficult.

Other countries across the world have a much more positive outlook on marijuana. Though illegal in more countries than not, quite a few places around the world have decriminalized or begun to tolerate the use of marijuana. For example, it is legal in Spain and Uruguay and decriminalized in the Virgin Islands, Ukraine, Switzerland, Slovenia, Russia, Portugal, the Netherlands and several other countries.

Laws on Cannabis

Laws concerning THC and CBD distribution are pretty sticky, to put it mildly. In the United States especially, there is a lot of confusion among lawmakers over the effects of marijuana. In states where medical marijuana has been legalized, it is generally only CBD that patients can use. There is still a heavy resistance to THC because of its psychoactive properties. Because of this, there are still state legislations that are against the use of CBD because they believe it may contain trace amounts of THC (the cutoff is 0.3 percent THC or less). However, even if it did, those trace amounts would have little to no psychoactive effect on users, but it shows that the United States is still hanging on to some of the same viewpoints from the war on drugs era.

Because there is such a hang-up on the psychoactive side of THC, many medical applications are denied in the preliminary stages. CBD-only treatments are often not as effective for many users as they would be paired with THC. These two cannabinoids are like a power couple; they work best together. For example, California scientists determined through their research that THC and CBD together had a stronger anti-tumoral effect than just CBD alone. Clinical research also showed that the two molecules together work better on neuropathic pain than either one on their own. It's unfortunate that a mild euphoric sensation from THC is viewed as a negative side effect when it contains so many health benefits.

Legislators often pass CBD-only laws but then make it nearly impossible for anyone to actually obtain the medicines by making it illegal to transport CBD over state lines. So even if a patient with a qualifying disorder (which, apart from Florida and Georgia, only includes intractable epilepsy and seizure disorders) finds a CBD medication that works for them, they may still be forced to commit a federal offense just to get it home. There is also an application process for patients to get a medical pass to purchase the cannabis they need, and after all that it only applies in the state in which they are listed as a medical user.

London-based pharmaceuticals have been working on a cannabidiol treatment for two very difficult forms of epilepsy, especially in children. As of December 2016, they were making progress on submitting it to the FDA and launching it commercially. If successfully accepted by the FDA, cannabis would need to be rescheduled from a Schedule 1 drug in order for patients in the US to get the much-needed prescriptions. But later that month the DEA took it one step further in the opposite direction; now all extracts (which includes CBD) are listed as a Schedule 1 drug. As stated earlier, Schedule 1 drugs are classified as having "no medical use," which is very clearly not the case for cannabis, especially CBD oils. Around the world, CBD is generally accepted in medical practices but recreational cannabis still faces deliberation.

The Big Deal About THC

THC (tetrahydrocannabinol) is a chemical compound, or cannabinoid, found in cannabis plants. It is regarded as the most psychoactive compound in marijuana. In simpler terms, Thorsten Rudroff, Ph.D. says, "...THC gives you the high feeling. The more THC you have, the more powerful the high." The other symptoms, such as increased appetite, relaxed feelings, and euphoria, are also caused by THC.

This compound produces these effects as it interacts with neurons in the brain. These neurons are able to communicate with each other through neurotransmitters, chemicals that deliver messages from one neuron to another by crossing the gaps and attaching to receptor molecules. This is how the brain communicates everything within the body. There is a particular neurotransmitter called an endocannabinoid. This one is important because it is very similar to cannabinoids in marijuana, both in appearance and functionality. Normally, endocannabinoids are released when the body experiences pain or stress, both physical and emotional, and work within the endocannabinoid system to relieve the pain. Cannabinoids in marijuana, such as THC, sneak into this system and attach themselves to the cannabinoid receptors.

There are two known types of cannabinoid receptors: CB1 and CB2. CB1 receptors are found in the learning, memory, anxiety, pain, and movement areas of the brain. When cannabinoids find their way to these receptors they throw off the regular functions of the endocannabinoid system, the one that relieves pain. Because the system is knocked off its regular course, the effects of marijuana can vary widely, from feeling stress relief to clumsiness to hunger cravings.

Essentially, THC increases the level of dopamine in the brain. Dopamine is a neurotransmitter that functions in the brain's reward and pleasure centers. It works, in part, to help the brain recognize "rewards" and seek them out. When THC meets a CB1 receptor and interacts with it, calcium is released from the neuron, causing it to stop functioning. When this neuron isn't working, it can't release its inhibitory molecule. These inhibitory molecules regulate the amount of dopamine in the brain. In other words, THC interacting with CB1 receptors leads to excess dopamine levels and heightened senses. This is what is known as a "high."

What About CBD?

Cannabidiol, or CBD, is another active compound found in marijuana. It is usually referred to along with THC as a sort of dynamic duo. CBD is known to have more sedative effects, and has been the main source of medical research. Because it's been discovered to have benefits on treating epilepsy and other neurological disorders, more and more research has been done to examine its effects on the brain in detail. CBD is unique in its potential for medicinal uses because it can affect a large number of brain and body receptors, including more than just cannabinoid receptors.

To know why CBD's versatility is important, the purpose of receptors must be understood. In the brain, neurons are connected by structures known as synapses. In these structures, neurons communicate with each other by sending neurotransmitters, or chemical messengers. To properly receive a message through a neurotransmitter, a neuron needs to have a receptor that fits it. When neurotransmitters can fit, or match, one of these receptors, then the neuron is capable of interacting directly with the messenger. Neurons contain various different receptors for neurotransmitters. Because CBD can affect so many different receptors, it has the ability to interact with all sorts of messages that the brain sends.

Most recent research has classified CBD as a negative allosteric modulator of the CB1 receptor. (The CB1 receptor is what THC interacts with to create excess levels of dopamine and the resulting high.) What this means is that CBD can bond to the same receptor in a different spot, and when it bonds at the same time that THC meets the receptor, the neuron that's affected gets a weaker signal. As stated before, THC affects the neuron to stop regulating dopamine levels. When the two cannabinoids react on the same receptor, the effect is much different than THC alone. Thus, CBD has become known for its ability to counteract the strong psychoactive effects of THC.

CBD and its medical benefits come from its effect on other receptors in the brain. It provides a therapeutic effect when it interacts with the TRPV-1 receptor. This is also known as the "vanilloid receptor", named after the vanilla bean which contains an essential oil with analgesic and antiseptic properties (pain-relieving and the ability to reduce likelihood of infection). When CBD binds with this receptor, it works as a stimulant to activate its abilities to regulate pain, inflammation, and body temperature. This is why cannabis with high levels of CBD works to treat neuropathic pain.

In higher concentrations, CBD can also activate the 5-HT1A serotonin receptor. This receptor is directly involved with biological processes relating to anxiety, sleep, pain, appetite, and more. When CBD interacts with 5-HT1A, it slows down its signaling and in turn ends up providing an antidepressant effect. In addition, CBD's anti-anxiety properties are due to its role on the adenosine receptor in the brain. These receptors regulate cardiovascular functions and have anti-inflammatory effects.

Though it activates the aforementioned receptors, CBD also provides medical benefits by deactivating the GPR55 receptor. It's involved in regulating blood pressure, bone density, and various other processes. When activated, GPR55 promotes the spread of cancer cells. Research done at the Chinese Academy of Sciences in Shanghai has shown this receptor expressed in several forms of cancer. Because CBD deactivates this receptor and blocks its signaling, it is believed to prevent the proliferation of cancer cells.

There are other ways in which CBD exerts anticancer effects. On every cell's nucleus there are PPARs (peroxisome proliferator activated receptors) that regulate energy maintenance, metabolic functions, and specifically proliferation of cells. When PPARs are activated, especially the PPAR-gamma receptor, proliferation is inhibited. Simply put, cancer cells are slowed down.

CBD and THC: How They Coexist

Clearly CBD and THC are very different cannabinoids. To sum it up, the biggest difference between the two is that THC is psychoactive and CBD is not. They both work within the body's endocannabinoid system, but CBD primarily interacts with the immune system and THC mainly causes reactions within the nervous system. Because the two compounds activate different receptors in the brain and nervous system, they initiate different symptoms in the body. According to an article from the British Journal of Pharmacology, THC is an agonist of CB1 and CB2 receptors, while CBD remains an antagonist of the same receptors, therefore causing a different physiological response. Because it doesn't interact directly with cannabinoid receptors, it does not have the psychoactive effects of THC.

CBD is known to combat some of the effects of THC. Instead of reacting directly with cannabinoid receptors in the way that THC does, CBD works to stop the enzyme that metabolizes anandamide, a natural cannabinoid found within the body. In turn, the release of dopamine and the effects that go along with it are stalled. CBD also promotes the release of another cannabinoid in the body that activates the same CB1 and CB2 receptors. What all of this means is that CBD and THC have similar pharmacological properties, but one works without causing a "high."

Researchers have noted this detail and many believe that CBD may actually help to counteract the intoxicating effects of THC and other psychotic symptoms. A recent study from the World Journal of Biological Psychiatry notes that more larger-scale studies need to be done before coming to hard conclusions, but there is evidence out there that CBD does possess several health properties, including acting as an antioxidant and antipsychotic. Though CBD is not known for its euphoric effects, cannabis with both THC and CBD present is still psychoactive.

Other Components of Marijuana

Though they get the most attention, THC and CBD are not the only active components in marijuana. There are over 80 active cannabinoids found in marijuana, but there are several to take note of. Cannabinol, or CBN, is an oxidation product of THC. Of all the known cannabinoids, CBN has the strongest sedative effects. Naturally, it is great for treating insomnia. CBG (cannabigerol) is another important cannabinoid. Though this one does not have the intoxicating effects of THC, it is said to be a crucial part of the whole psychoactive cycle. CBC (cannabichromene) is similar, but primarily important for reducing anxiety and stress.

In addition to cannabinoids, there are active components known as terpenes. These are "flavors" that impact any high. There are five terpenes that influence all strains of cannabis in varying levels: myrcene, limonene, pinene, linalool, and terpinolene. Myrcene has one of the biggest effects on a high, while delivering hints of minty, tropical, and earthy aromas. Limonene is often sought after in strains because it allows more THC to reach the brain and adds very pleasant notes of citrus. Pinene has flavors of pine, rosemary, and sage in the strains in which it's more concentrated and promotes stronger memory and alertness. Linalool delivers a floral scent reminiscent of lavender, and when combined with terpinolene or limonene it can be sweet like candy. Terpinolene, thus, can be sweet and citrusy, but primarily it delivers a fresh, woody, herbal aroma.

Indica, Sativa, and Hybrids: What's the Difference?

Though there are countless strains of cannabis, there are several categories that are important to know: indica, sativa, and hybrid. Most strains of marijuana can be grouped into one of these three classifications, and each has their own set of properties. When shopping for a certain effect or flavor, there is a way to distinguish indica from sativa simply by appearance. Pure sativa plants grow taller with thinner leaves and smaller buds. In general, sativa originates from Southeast Asia, India, regions of Africa, Indochina, and Northeastern India; the plants grow best in warm, humid climates. On the other hand, indica grows into a much shorter and wider plant with larger, fanned leaves and denser buds. They thrive in drier climates in Central and Southern Asia, particularly Pakistan, Afghanistan, and India. These plants can also produce unique red and blue hues when exposed to the cold, which can be another way to determine the strain.

In addition to their physical appearances, indica and sativa strains are known for their different effects. In a nutshell, indica is known to have more calming, sedative effects and delivers a full-body high. Sometimes this is referred to as "couch-lock" by frequent users. Sativa tends to be better for those who want to maintain their energy, and its high is primarily cerebral. This is a more ideal strain for creativity. According to a poll on Leafly. com, users rated their experiences between an indica strain "Bubba Kush" and a sativa "Sour Diesel." Bubba Kush left users feeling primarily relaxed, happy, and sleepy. Sour Diesel had different effects; the top 3 experiences were happy, euphoric, and uplifted.

For medicinal purposes, both strains can be helpful. For fatigue or depression, sativa strains are more popular. It can also be helpful with ADD or mood disorders. A more relaxing strain of indica is generally better for pain or insomnia.

As far as THC and CBD content, an overly simplified answer is that indica features a higher THC:CBD ratio and sativa claims a higher CBD:THC ratio. This explanation is based on a theory from Leaf Science that high THC plants have genes that code for the enzyme

THCA synthase. This enzyme induces a chemical reaction that creates THCA, which will become THC when exposed to heat. The plants with this quality are usually indica. However, this is just one theory. It's not exactly that simple. When it comes down to it, smokeable cannabis in general will contain high levels of THC. What causes the varying effects between indica, sativa, and hybrids depends heavily on the kinds of terpenes (fragrant oils that are found in plants and herbs including cannabis) found and the concentrations of those.

Hybrids are, naturally, combinations of the strains. In other words, hybrids can show dominance from either the indica or sativa side or be a balance of both. When growers mix genetics from differing regions, a hybrid is born. These can be extremely useful for those who are looking for specific benefits, such as a creative high that relaxes the body enough to relieve pain.

Marijuana Strains

Breeding cannabis is not a new idea, as early on, humans started changing the plant based on ever-evolving needs. But the popularity of breeding "customized" cannabis has increased exponentially in the modern era for a number of reasons. Ever since the prohibition of marijuana, breeding cannabis for shorter flowering times, higher potencies, and greater yields became a central focus. This was a central goal in order to successfully sell marijuana on the black market. As time went on, the recreational cannabis industry flourished and growers have been taking advantage of new technologies and customer requests to get creative with their strains.

This pro-marijuana community has come together despite laws and stigma largely in part to online forums. High Times and Leafly are examples of popular websites where users can go to meet other people with similar opinions, gain knowledge, and keep up to date on the latest cannabis news. The Cannabis Cup is another opportunity for the recreational industry to grow; Cannabis

Cup is a trade show nearly thirty years in practice that showcases the latest developments in all things marijuana. Because of this ever-growing community, growers are seeing opportunity to meet people's various needs and desires in their weed strains.

Different strains are bred for various purposes; they vary in aroma, flavor, potency, medical purpose, side effects, etc. They are generally named based on the growers and/or by the smell, color, or flavor of the strain. Though there are countless varieties of cannabis, there are several ways to group them together. The easiest way to differentiate between groups of strains is with these three classifications: indica, sativa, and hybrid. As stated before, indica strains generally have a similar sedative effect while sativas are generally better for higher energy and alertness. Hybrids can show a balanced effect or lean way or the other. As marijuana has become increasingly less taboo, growers have begun to turn their focus away from breeding strains for potency and higher yields and toward cultivating new flavors and terpenoid content. It has become an art.

Though the number of existing strains would be impossible to count as there are new strains developed constantly, there are definitely some that have stood out for consumers. In 2015, the following strains ranked most popular:

* * *

Gorilla Glue #4	Sunset Sherbet
Critical Kush	Tangie
Candyland	Jedi Kush
ACDC	Animal Cookies
Bubblegum Kush	OG #18

* * *

The top ranking, Gorilla Glue #4, had a 906% increase in user ratings and reviews. This unique blend provides users with a relaxed, extremely euphoric high. Its aroma is potent, earthy, and definitely lends truth to the "skunky" stereotype of weed smells. Critical Kush is an indica strain that was born from mixing OG Kush and Critical Mass, two already popular strains. It's high in THC but comes with a CBD profile that balances the effects to provide a high similar to a "slow massage," according to a user. Candyland got its name from its uniquely sweet flavor, and the buds are colored blue, green, white, and purple. Not only is it beautiful to look at but its effects are very pleasant, both uplifting and calming. ACDC is 4th on the list and the first high-CBD strain in this collection. This one has been rated great for medical patients because it provides a potent high that chases away pain without the cerebral effects or any haziness. It also delivers lemony notes, which is a unique property; many high-CBD strains have a grassy fragrance that may be unpleasant to many users.

This new approach to breeding marijuana plants has definitely helped pave the way for more medical marijuana strains. Depending on the treatment desired, growers can evaluate different strains and their benefits and then work to combine them for the most potent therapeutic strains. Those benefitting from medical marijuana may use a combination of strains. Since sativas induce a more alert, energetic high with heightened creativity, a patient suffering from fatigue or depression would benefit from using this strain during the daytime. However, this would not be the best choice for that patient at nighttime. Indica strains come in at this time, offering a full-body sedative effect and aiding a more restful sleep. For people with anxiety, indica may be best during the day.

Hybrids can offer the best of both. A popular hybrid is Blue Dream, which is sativa-dominant. Its sativa influences means that it provides an uplifting high, but when balanced with an indica strain it gives a full-body high while maintaining the cerebral effects. It's a perfect example of a strain best for patients suffering from pain, depression, or nausea. These ailments require a high THC strain, which can result in side effects that make it difficult to go about the day. Blue Dream relieves pain and nausea while still allowing patients to be productive and alert.

Marijuana Concentrates

When it comes to consuming marijuana, most people have a certain image that comes to mind. It most likely involves a joint, a blunt, or a pipe to smoke out of. Some may think of pot brownies. But there is so much more to the marijuana experience. More experienced users have leapt into the world of cannabis concentrates: hash, oils, kief, rosin, and other variations. These concentrates are often preferred because they are more potent. This can suit both the recreational user and the medical patient; more potent cannabis, in the form of a concentrate, will cause a greater high or greater medical benefits with smaller amounts.

Using cannabis concentrates is not a new idea. Hash, in particular, has been cultivated for thousands of years. Hash is cannabis flower that has had its plant material and the resinous trichomes mechanically separated. There are several ways to go about this separation process. "Dry sifting" is a method where the flower is separated by hand through sieves or tumblers. The method is comparable to grinding weed before packing a bowl. The resulting fine powder, or "kief," is then pressed into hash with the use of heat. "Ice-water separation" (resulting in "iceolator", which has very high THC content) is another way to make hash. The idea is that through agitation and ice water, the more resinous pieces of the cannabis flower will sink to the bottom and the excess inactive plant parts will stay floating toward the top. The iceolator hash that's produced is a very pure form and will contain no solvent residues.

Hash is quality checked in a number of ways. Firstly, color is important. In a dry sifting method, the resulting kief will be more golden in color if it is more pure. When it's green, that means there is still some contamination from plant material. The resulting brick of hash should have a dark, shiny surface that shows the active trichomes have melted together. Hash should also light easily and give off a pure odor. Any chemical smells are a bad sign. It should also leave a white ash, which indicates purity. For hand rolled hash, it should be soft and sticky on the inside when the brick is broken.

Shatter, budder, and oil are terms that may be unfamiliar for some. Shatter, the most potent, is a form of cannabis concentrate that resembles peanut brittle in appearance; it should have a smooth, clear finish. Oil resembles honey in appearance. It can be hard to work with because of its sticky consistency. Budder is creamier, bearing resemblance to the mixture of sugar and butter whipped together. Each of these concentrates can be used with the same devices, such as vape pens or oil rigs, but there are different benefits to each. Though shatter is the most potent at potentially 80% THC, it can lack the terpenes that give ordinary marijuana its taste and aroma. Budder is usually around 70% THC but still retains some of the terpenes and is more flavorful. Oil is the most flavorful and the least potent.

Rosin and BHO are two other terms to make note of. BHO, or "butane hash oil," is cannabis concentrate that is extracted by using butane as a solvent. Shatter, budder, and oil can all be classified as forms of BHO. Rosin, on the other hand, does not require the butane solvent. It is a concentrate that can actually be made without any solvents. All that's required is heat and pressure to get the resinous oil out from the flowers or buds. It's such a simple process that one can even do it at home with heat from a standard hair straightener. Rosin looks much like other forms of concentrates, such as shatter, but it's preferred by many because it lacks any residual solvents that other forms of cannabis extract have due to their extraction processes.

Where to Find It

Legal dispensaries sell most of their marijuana products, even topical applications, containing both THC and CBD. However, conflicting and confusing laws make it hard for users to know what they can or cannot buy, grow, or distribute.

The state of Colorado remains the epitome of marijuana acceptance. The law states that adults 21 and older can possess up to one ounce of marijuana and consume legally. You do not have to be a Colorado resident to purchase and use within state borders. But it's important to note that when purchasing, there are some guidelines in place for how much you can mix and match between flowers and concentrates. Though it's legal to consume, there is still implied discretion. In other words, walking down the street and lighting a blunt is not generally accepted. It's similar to open-container laws with alcohol.

There is also regulation on driving under the influence of THC.

Amsterdam has also held extremely open views of cannabis use for years now. While recreational drugs are still technically illegal here, soft drugs (such as cannabis and hashish) have been severely decriminalized. The general outlook is protecting the health and safety of Dutch residents, and thus there is a much more logical opinion of marijuana in place. Coffee shops that allow the purchase and open use of cannabis and other soft drugs are generally left alone if they do not cause any disturbances. Dutch laws target much more harshly the trafficking of recreational drugs. Spain also uses the idea of "Cannabis Clubs", where users can openly smoke and partake in the use of cannabis, and public consumption is also decriminalized, though there are still fines and other standard laws in place to regulate this.

In states such as Arizona where medical marijuana is legalized, patients still must apply for a medical card. In order to purchase medical marijuana, a patient must be at least 18 years old, have at least one of the conditions on the approved list (in Arizona the conditions include cancer, glaucoma, hepatitis C, and Crohn's disease), find and schedule an appointment with a specific medical marijuana doctor, and then submit the application and wait for a card. Once approved, patients can go to any state-licensed dispensaries for their cannabis products.

Purchasing from dispensaries is not as simple as walking into a grocery store and walking out. As shown in a dispensary tour on the Weedmaps YouTube channel, there is a process for admitting patients into some dispensaries. This particular video highlighted South Coast Caregivers in Santa Ana, California. Medical papers are required before filling out the additional paperwork that is specific to this dispensary. There is a waiting room that patients must pass through before being let into the main product room, where volunteers assist with finding the right strains, forms, and tools for each customer.

There have been definite improvements in clearing the taboo on cannabis, but there's still a large amount of work to be done.

What THC and CBD Can Do For our Health

THC

Many studies have been conducted to dig deeper into the medical benefits of THC. Evidence has shown that people suffering from chronic pain, nausea, lack of appetite, and stress have greatly benefited from the effects of THC. This cannabinoid works to alleviate pain by activating pathways in the central nervous system that block pain signals. Specifically, it has been shown to aid in reducing nerve-related pain. A study conducted on patients suffering from neuropathic pain with little to no help from other treatments showed that they experienced relief with low doses of cannabis. It can also help with stress and anxiety when it interacts with the amygdala in the brain. The amygdala governs emotional responses, such as fear and anxiety. THC can change this response for the better. Particularly in people who have a shortage of endocannabinoids (neurotransmitters that relieve

pain) due to past traumas or excess stress, THC can re-
plenish these amounts and provide therapeutic relief.
Though sometimes THC can overstimulate the amygdala and cause feelings of paranoia or heightened anxiety,
this usually only happens when a variety of other factors
are in place: consuming exceedingly high amounts of
THC, being in unfamiliar surroundings, or mixing other
drugs or alcohol with marijuana. When consumed without these factors, there is extremely low risk for negative
effects.

Both THC and CBD are used in medical applications, but each has different properties that work best for
certain ailments. In short, THC has the following effects:

❑ Relaxation

❑ Sleepiness

❑ Increased appetite

❑ Increased levels of calm

❑ Altered senses (sight, smell, hearing)

Because of these effects, it has proven effective in a number of ways in the medical field. It can help counteract the side effects of chemotherapy, primarily reducing nausea and promoting a healthy appetite. In other diseases where loss of appetite is prevalent, such as AIDS, THC can definitely make a difference. For spinal injuries, multiple sclerosis, and other muscular disorders, it's helpful for lessening spasms and tremors and alleviating pain.

CBD

CBD oil specifically is the subject of many medical studies. Project CBD is a website and non-profit organization that devotes its time to promoting healthy awareness about the true medical benefits of cannabidiol. What's great about cannabidiol is that it is extremely safe. A study published on PubMed revealed that cannabidiol is non-toxic is non-transformed cells. Studies also show that it does not alter psychomotor or psychological functions. Plus, chronic use and high doses (up to 1,500 mg/day) have shown to be easily tolerated by humans.

CBD has the following effects:

- ❑ Anxiety relief

- ❑ Decreased inflammation

- ❑ Counteracting psychotic symptoms

- ❑ Nausea relief

CBD can help to treat many similar issues that THC can, including the negative side effects that go along with chemotherapy. It can also support healthy appetite and suppress vomiting and nausea. On the other hand, it improves the range for cannabis in the medical field by working with a number of different disorders that cause high levels of anxiety. Depression, social anxiety, and schizophrenia are just several disorders that can be easier to deal with by using CBD. Depressive symptoms, anxiety, paranoia, and many other psychotic symptoms can be alleviated this way.

Generally, CBD is much more widely accepted in the medical field. This is because it lacks the intoxicating effects of THC, which can become too much for some people. It's also rated extremely safe according to a number of studies. Research has shown that CBD does not have a negative effect on embryonic cells, motor skills, blood pressure, or heart rate. So while it works to give many people comfort, there's little risk of negative side effects.

In many instances, finding the perfect ratio of THC and CBD in medical marijuana delivers the best result. For example, one might need the appetite-stimulating effects of THC but also need their symptoms of anxiety reduced with CBD. One condition that would require a combination of THC and CBD is chronic obstructive pulmonary disease (COPD). Its symptoms include coughing, shortness of breath, wheezing, and clogged airways. This disease is also progressive, meaning that it gets worse over time. In this case, CBD would help considerably with reducing inflammation while THC and its relaxing effect could soothe and relax constricted airways.

Consuming Cannabis

Smoking marijuana is the most common way to use. It's easy because it requires little tools or extra preparation, and smoking provides fast results. When a user smokes, the effects of the cannabinoids hit the bloodstream quickly and cause their intended effects almost right away. People have been smoking marijuana since 2,500 BC (though the Western Hemisphere did not catch on until around the 1800s).

However, smoking in general does have some negative side effects. Smoking can damage the lungs over time, which is a well-known fact. Often times people will combine marijuana and tobacco while smoking, and it's commonly known that tobacco consumption causes negative side effects. Tobacco can cause cancer, respiratory conditions, fertility issues, and more. Though cannabis alone will cause none of these effects (and is known to in fact have anticancer properties), smoking is likely the least healthy way to use. This is for several reasons.

First, users who smoke marijuana will inhale more

smoke and generally hold it longer than any tobacco user would with cigarettes. Secondly, if the user is smoking from joints or blunts they are inhaling more than just the cannabis flower inside. The blunt wraps are often made of tobacco themselves. Though there is not a lot of evidence that smoking pure marijuana causes serious detrimental damage to the lungs, there are still chemicals in marijuana smoke that can be harmful, such as carbon monoxide or hydrogen cyanide. The point to be made, though, is that these harmful chemicals come from burning the plant material itself and not the active cannabinoids in marijuana. So consuming marijuana in other ways would not release these chemicals.

When deciding how to use marijuana for medical purposes, there are healthier options. As discussed earlier, smoking is one of the least healthy ways to use marijuana. And it makes no sense to smoke for a lot of medical patients, especially if they are using marijuana for respiratory issues. To get around this issue, vaporizing has become a popular method. Vaporization of concentrates and extracts produces less harmful carcinogens, such as tar and ammonia, than typical marijuana or tobacco smoke. Because of the higher temperature required to vaporize marijuana, less smoke is produced and more cannabinoids can be extracted. Thus, it is more effective and efficient. There's also much less odor with vaporization, making this an ideal option for medical patients who want or need to exercise discretion.

Edibles are also an excellent and discreet option for medical users. Obviously, there is no smoke or odor involved when consuming an edible. This is handy for users where oral intake is an easier method of medication, and there's the added benefit that consuming edibles doesn't have quite the same stigma that smoking weed does for medical purposes. Many people can't get behind the idea that someone would smoke something for medicine, so for those in conservative communities edibles are the best way to avoid judgment. And with the ever-advancing edible culture, people can consume their cannabis in more ways than the stereotypical pot brownie. Soup broths, fruit, trail mix, desserts, and other healthy snacks have found their way into the edible category. This way, especially for medical patients, there's no need to sacrifice other aspects of their health just to consume medication.

There is a vast variety of edibles, and they account for nearly half of the cannabis industry revenue. Edible marijuana can be found in candies (fruit gummies, suckers, or chocolate), health foods (nuts, fruits, granola bars), or even extra flavorings and condiments to add to your existing dishes (honey, butter, etc.). There is no limit to edible creativity. For example, the 2016 NorCal Medical Cannabis Cup edible entries included macaroons, cereal bars, sugar-free chocolate, bacon, and barbecue sauce.

There are a variety of ways to make edibles, but a popular route to go is to make "canna-butter" or marijuana-infused butter that can be used in place of regular butter in whatever recipes you desire. This is done using a double-boiler. The marijuana is ground, wrapped in cheesecloth, and secured with cooking twine to make a pouch that can sit in a mixture of melted butter and water in the top part of the boiler. At the end of the process, the cannabis and melted butter solution is chilled and the water is left at the bottom with a solid mass of canna-butter at the top. This kind of process can be done with many food items and can be done at home on a small-scale.

When edibles are made in licensed kitchens, there are very strict guidelines and regulations that come into play. Only approved chefs can work in the kitchen and there are strict portion control rules. There are also potency regulations and testing that edibles must go through in order to get proper labels and product information before being sold in dispensaries.

There are also many topical applications for cannabis. The benefits of using cannabis topically are administering targeted relief through the skin, the body's largest organ, without the neurological effects. Particularly, indica strains are used most often in topical applications because they provide the best relief for physical symptoms. Topical marijuana is used for eczema, psoriasis, arthritic pain, and even some skin infections.

The Future of Cannabis

The idea of marijuana being legal and openly accepted across the world may be a futuristic ideal, but it is not impossible. Though medical research has to overcome many obstacles to dig deeper and publish more studies on the health benefits of marijuana, the recreational cannabis community is sure to keep growing and gaining members. As the younger generations continue to grow up with an open-minded view of this natural herb, there is hope that society will be able to learn and unleash all of marijuana's practical uses and possible benefits. In the meantime, enjoy this tasty recipe for peanut butter cookies that pack an extra punch.

Punchy Peanut Butter Cookies

Yields:

About 30 cookies

Ingredients:

1 cup canna-butter (recipe to follow)

1 cup sugar

1 cup creamy peanut butter

1 large egg

2 ½ cups all-purpose flour

¼ tsp salt

2 tsp vanilla extract

Instructions

1. Preheat oven to 350 degrees.
2. Combine canna-butter, peanut butter, salt, and sugar in a large mixing bowl and beat until fluffy.
3. Add egg and vanilla extract.
4. Add flour and mix until you get an evenly mixed dough.
5. Lightly grease a cookie sheet.
6. Divide dough into golf-ball sized balls and place 2-3 inches apart on sheet, flattening them with a floured hand.
7. Bake for 7-9 minutes or until golden brown.

Canna-Butter

Ratio:

1 oz weed for 2 cups butter

Instructions

1. Fill a pot with about 1-2 inches of water and bring to a boil.
2. Add butter.
3. When butter is melted, turn heat to low and add ground marijuana buds.
4. Simmer for at least 3 hours.
5. Let cool.
6. Using cheesecloth and a bowl, filter out plant material. Place cannabis and butter mixture in cheesecloth and squeeze as much liquid out as possible into the bowl beneath.
7. Set aside the drained plant material. Place the rest of the mixture into the fridge to chill for at least 30 minutes.
8. When the mixture is ready you'll see that the butter and cannabis will have hardened in the bowl and the water will be separated. Skim the butter from the top of the water and place in new container.
9. Toss the water after you've removed all the butter and place the new butter back in the fridge until ready to use.

Enjoy!

Bonus

Welcome to HMPL Publishing! Let's start right away with an exclusive bonus made available only for our inner circle.

Get your free eBook **'The best DIY THC & CBD recipes to prepare at home'** here: http://eepurl.com/cx-pVZf

Subscribing to our newsletter will get you the latest THC and CBD recipes, articles and some of our upcoming eBooks for absolutely free. To make that even better we'll update you with the most recent information about marijuana, medical breakthroughs, and the various applications of cannabis.

You can visit also http://happyhealthygreen.life

Or connect with us on Facebook;
https://www.facebook.com/happyhealthygreen.life

Sources Used

This is a list of all the titles of the researches used for this book. You may look them up by searching the full title of the research on Google as most of them are publically available.

Bacca, Angela. "What's the Difference Between Hemp and Marijuana?" *Alternet,* 5 June 2014. http://www.alternet.org/drugs/whats-difference-between-hemp-and-marijuana

Bergamaschi, MM, et al. "Safety and side effects of cannabidiol, a Cannabis sativa constituent." *Current Drug Safety,* 1 September 2011. https://www.ncbi.nlm.nih.gov/pubmed/22129319

"The Best Hashish in Amsterdam?! How to Test the Quality of Your Hash." *Smokers Guide,* 2016. https://www.smokersguide.com/quotes/55/the_best_hashish_in_amsterdam___how_to_test_the_qu.html#.WJ3drBLytPM

"Busted: America's War on Marijuana." *PBS,* 2014. http://www.pbs.org/wgbh/pages/frontline/shows/dope/etc/cron.html

"*Cannabis sativa* L. marijuana." *USDA Natural Resources Conservation Service.* https://plants.usda.gov/core/profile?symbol=casa3

"Cannabis Craftsmanship: How to Make Hash." *YouTube,* uploaded by Leafly, 18 December 2015. https://www. youtube.com/watch?v=aGm1Ssq9u2s

"Concentrate Basics: Shatter, Budder and Oil." *YouTube,* uploaded by High Times, 27 May 2014. https://www. youtube.com/watch?v=zbAY763zt4M

"Drug Schedules." *Drug Enforcement Administration,* 2017. https://www.dea.gov/druginfo/ds.shtml

"Drugs Policy in the Netherlands." *UKCIA,* 1997. http:// www.ukcia.org/research/dutch.php

Eisinger, Amy. "Here's What Actually Happens When You Smoke Weed." *Greatist,* 13 October 2016. http://greatist. com/health/your-brain-on-marijuana

"The Health Effects of Cannabis and Cannabinoids: The Current State of Evidence and Recommendations for Research." *The National Academies of Sciences, Engineering, and Medicine,* 12 January 2017. http:// nationalacademies.org/hmd/reports/2017/health-effects-of-cannabis-and-cannabinoids.aspx

"Health Effects of Cigarette Smoking." *Centers for Disease Control and Prevention,* 1 December 2016. https://www. cdc.gov/tobacco/data_statistics/fact_sheets/health_effects/ effects_cig_smoking/index.htm

High Times, 2017. http://hightimes.com/

High Times Cannabis Cup, 2015. https://www.cannabiscup. com/

Hoey, Dennis. "As Mainers celebrate legal marijuana, where does new law draw the line?" *Portland Press Herald,* 30 January 2017. http://www.pressherald.com/2017/01/30/legal-marijuana-celebrated-by-maine-businesses-advocates/?platform=hootsuite

Hoff, Tom. "What decriminalized cannabis looks like in Spain." *Students for Sensible Drug Policy,* 31 March 2014. http://ssdp.org/news/blog/what-decriminalized-cannabis-looks-like-in-spain/

"How CBD Works." *Project CBD,* 2017. https://www.projectcbd.org/how-cbd-works

"How Does CBD Affect the Endocannabinoid System?" *CBD Oil Review,* 2015. https://cbdoilreview.org/cbd-cannabidiol/cbd-endocannabinoid-system/

Khoury, JM, et al. "Is there a role for cannabidiol in psychiatry?" *The World Journal of Biological Psychiatry,* 23 January 2017. https://www.ncbi.nlm.nih.gov/pubmed/28112021

Leafly, 2017. https://www.leafly.com/

Leaf Science, 2017. http://www.leafscience.com/

"Legality of cannabis by country." *Wikipedia,* 13 February 2017. https://en.wikipedia.org/wiki/Legality_of_cannabis_by_country

"Legality of Cannabis." *Wikipedia,* 10 February 2017. https://en.wikipedia.org/wiki/Legality_of_cannabis

"Marijuana Intoxication." *MedlinePlus,* 13 January 2015. https://medlineplus.gov/ency/article/000952.htm

"Marijuana Laws in Colorado." *Pot Guide,* 2016. https://www.coloradopotguide.com/marijuana-laws-in-colorado/

"Marijuana vs Tobacco Smoke Compositions." *National Academy Press,* 1988. https://erowid.org/plants/cannabis/cannabis_info3.shtml

Niesink, Raymond J.M. and Margriet W. van Lear. "Does Cannabidiol Protect Against Adverse Psychological Effects of THC?" *Frontiers in Psychiatry,* 16 October 2013. https://www.ncbi.nlm.nih.gov/pmc/articles/PMC3797438/

Pardes, Arielle. "Marijuana Is Still a Schedule 1 Drug, Judge Rules." *Vice,* 15 April 2015. https://www.vice.com/en_us/article/marijuana-is-still-a-schedule-i-drug-judge-rules-415

Prichard, Ry. "Concentrates 101: What's on the market, from kief and CO2 oil to BHO." *The Cannabist,* 19 June 2015. http://www.thecannabist.co/2015/06/19/marijuana-concentrates-kief-bho-water-hash-co2-oil-wax-shatter/36386/

Project CBD, 2017. https://www.projectcbd.org/

Shapiro, Maren. "No High Risk: Marijuana May Be Less Harmful Than Alcohol, Tobacco." *NBC News,* 26 February 2015. http://www.nbcnews.com/storyline/legal-pot/no-high-risk-marijuana-may-be-less-harmful-alcohol-tobacco-n312876

"State Info, United States." *Norml*, 2017. http://norml.org/states

"THC vs CBD." *Medical Marijuana Journal*, 2 August 2013. http://www.mmjjournal.com/thc-vs-cbd/

"This Is How Pot Edibles Are Made." *YouTube*, uploaded by MSNBC, 22 December 2014. https://www.youtube.com/watch?v=jFV3Nb-ulSo

"Topical Use of Cannabis." *Cannabis Plus: Natural Alternatives for Health*. http://cannabisplus.net/topical-use-of-cannabis/

"What is COPD?" *National Heart, Lung, and Blood Institute*, 31 July 2013. https://www.nhlbi.nih.gov/health/health-topics/topics/copd/

"What is the Difference Between THC and CBD?" *CBD Oil Review*, 2015. https://cbdoilreview.org/cbd-cannabidiol/thc-cbd/

Wilsey, B., et al. "Low-dose vaporized cannabis significantly improves neuropathic pain." *The Journal of Pain*, Febuary 2013. https://www.ncbi.nlm.nih.gov/pubmed/23237736

"2016 NorCal Medical Cannabis Cup: Edible Entries." *YouTube*, uploaded by High Times, 17 June 2016. https://www.youtube.com/watch?v=wm0JyVbjq88